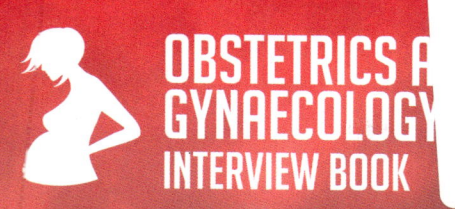

OBSTETRICS A... GYNAECOLOGY INTERVIEW BOOK

CONTENTS

1. PORTFOLIO STATION	1-21
2. CLINICAL STATION	22-46
3. COMMUNICATION STATION	47-72

PREFACE

The **Nepalese Doctors Association UK** (NDAUK) is one of the most prestigious organisations that has maintained the highest standards of professional integrity right from its inception in 1985, and has become a symbol of unity among doctors of Nepalese origin. We have on going inspiring projects to raise charity funds to help post earthquake reconstruction and rehabilitation in Nepal.

I am delighted to present this interview book, written by Dr Neha Shah and Dr Chawan Baran to you. The book provides a valuable resource for any doctor applying for Obstetric and Gynaecology specialty training. The charity fund raised by this project will go directly to buy more ambulances to transport sick and vulnerable patients in the remote eastern region of Taplejung, Nepal. For the first time in the history of NDA UK, we are dedicating a special preface in a book to acknowledge a significant contribution made by the authors.

MISS BEENA SUBBA
Consultant Obstetrician & Gynaecologist
MD, FRCOG
Chair, NDAUK

PORTFOLIO STATION
& MARK SCHEME

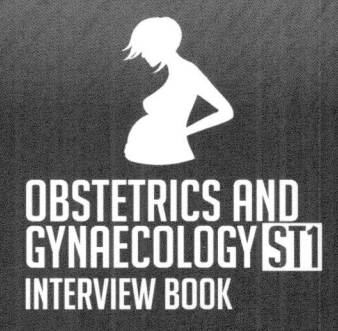

OBSTETRICS AND GYNAECOLOGY ST1 INTERVIEW BOOK

www.obsandgynae.net

PORTFOLIO STATION

Portfolio interview stations commonly cover four themes, which carry approximately equal weighting.

- Understanding of and commitment to the specialty
- Training priorities (for the first 12 months, and beyond)
- Quality improvement measures (including audit)
- Teaching and research

Interviewers are trying to ascertain your insight into the specialty, therefore it is important to speak to existing trainees, read the person specification and go through the RCOG website.

Each station is only about ten minutes long so there is not a lot of time to highlight your strengths. As such, it is imperative to be concise and time your answers appropriately. We recommend not spending more than one minute per answer, and to split your time equally between the above categories.

WHY OBSTETRICS AND GYNAECOLOGY?

This will probably be the first question you will be asked, so it is vital to have a specific and personalised answer to give yourself a good starting impression.

Example reasons:

- A diverse specialty encompassing acute management (e.g. labour ward), chronic management (e.g. gynaecology clinics), diagnostics of ultrasound and surgical management.
- Strong communication aspect.
- Surgical specialty.
- Diagnostics of ultrasound.
- Ability to make a significant difference to women's quality of life.
- Physiology of pregnancy fascinating.
- Multidisciplinary team approach.

WHAT WOULD YOUR TRAINING PRIORITIES BE IN THE FIRST 12 MONTHS?

- Achieve the basic competencies in the 19 core modules and complete other requirements needed to pass your Annual Review of Competence Progression (ARCP).
- Focus on obtaining labour ward experience.
- Pass MRCOG part 1.
- Develop basic ultrasound competencies (and attend an ultrasound course).
- By doing the above, develop the skills to be competent when second on call (ST3).

THE STRUCTURE OF THE TRAINING PROGRAMME

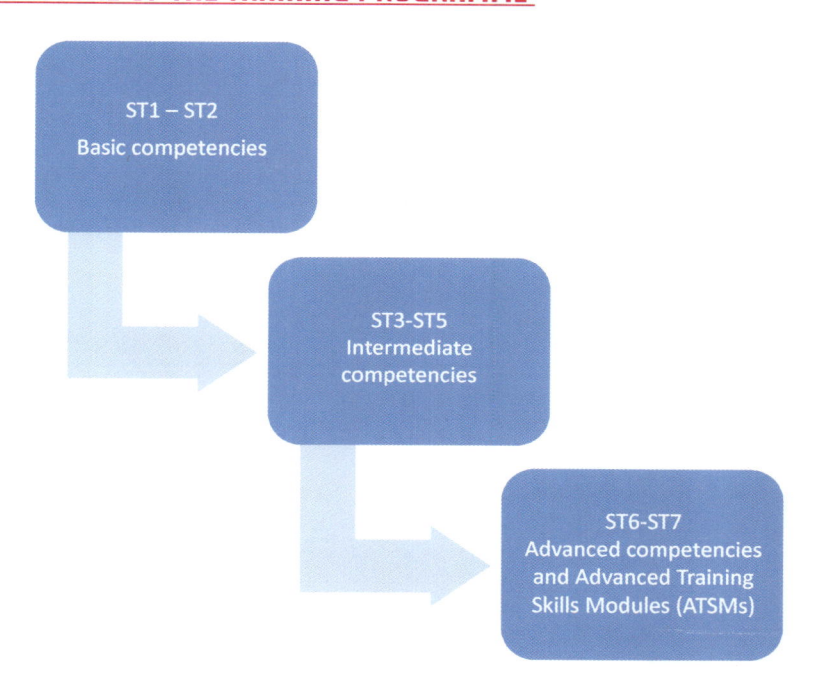

ST1 – ST2
Basic competencies

ST3-ST5
Intermediate competencies

ST6-ST7
Advanced competencies and Advanced Training Skills Modules (ATSMs)

ST1/ST2 COMPETENCIES

Procedures (OSATS - Objective Structured Assessment of Technical Skills)

- **Formative**
- Hysteroscopy
- Laparoscopy
- Basic ultrasound scanning

- **Summative**
- Basic Caesarean section
- Ventouse delivery
- Forceps delivery
- Foetal blood sampling
- Surgical management of miscarriage
- Manual removal of placenta
- Perineal repair

Courses

- Basic Practical Skills in Obstetrics and Gynaecology
- CTG Training
- Obstetric Simulation Course (e.g. PROMPT, ALSO)
- Basic ultrasound course
- Third degree tear course

Workplace Based Assessments

- 8 mini-CEXs (clinical evaulation exercises) per year
- 8 CBDs (case based discussions) per year
- 8 reflective practices per year

Examinations

- MRCOG part 1

Attendance

- 100% of available regional teaching
- Local risk management meeting

Other

- TO1s (Team observation) to be completed atleast twice a year
- One completed and presented clinical governance project per year
- Documented evidence of teaching
- Departmental presentation

REQUIREMENTS OF ST1

NOTES :

- Formative – shows evidence of training since last ARCP.
- Summative – shows competence (need at least 3 assessments by at least two difference assessors).

A recent change in the training pathway :
- There is a greater emphasis on ultrasound, with ultrasound competencies and attendance at a basic ultrasound course now being a requirement of ST1 and ST2.

THE FUTURE OF OBSTETRICS AND GYNAECOLOGY

- Shift towards 24-hour consultant-delivered care (versus consultant-led care).
- Centralisation of specialist services – e.g. endometriosis centres.
- Shift of workload to community – e.g. community gynaecology.
- Trend towards medical management of gynaecological conditions and therefore a reduction in surgical management (e.g. heavy menstrual bleeding was previously often managed by hysterectomy. Now there are a number of alternative medical options including mirena coil and endometrial ablation).
- Increase in the number of female trainees in the workforce – increase in part-time workers and maternity leave.
- Increasing maternal age at childbirth, thereby increasing co-morbidities in the obstetric population with a greater need to manage medical conditions in obstetrics.

TOP TIP:

When mentioning the shift towards 24-hour consultant delivered services, state that you understand this means as a consultant you will be working a shift pattern (including night shifts on-site) and you are willing to do so because:

1. Patient safety is your priority.
2. Although you will be working night shifts, you understand that you will be given compensatory time off.

TOP TIP:

When discussing the increase in co-morbidities in the obstetric population and the increasing emphasis on management of medical conditions in pregnancy, mention that this is highlighted by the MBRRACE report. The MBRRACE Maternal Mortality report 2015 shows that two thirds of maternal mortality is due to INDIRECT causes (deaths due to pre-existing medical conditions or mental health problems).

CHALLENGES FACING TRAINEES AND HOW TO OVERCOME THEM

Insufficient training opportunities (secondary to European Working Time Directive and reduced surgical workload)	Maximise training opportunities- workplace based assessments (WBA), eLearning, courses, simulation training, additional reading.
Fragmentation of care (secondary to European Working Time Directive)	Meticulous hand-over, be proactive in following up cases
Increased litigation	Accurate documentation, seek senior support when required, good communication skills

NOTES :

- Workplace Based Assessments include
- Case Based Discussions (CBDs)
- Clinical Evaluation Exercises (Mini-CEX)
- Objective Structured Assessment of Technical Skills (OSATs)

TELL US ABOUT YOUR TEACHING EXPERIENCE

- Use a maximum of three examples, covering a range of teaching styles (e.g. small group/large group, didactic/interactive, formal/informal, clinical/communication/practical skills).
- Discuss feedback received.
- Mention if you have had any formal teaching experience.
- When describing feedback
  - First mention positive feedback.
  - Then mention any negative feedback.
  - Finish by explaining how you have used that negative feedback to improve your teaching practice, thereby finishing on a positive note.

Examples of Positive Feedback

1) Clear and concise
2) Positive and encouraging
3) Sets appropriate goals
4) Involves students
5) Able to adapt to students level of knowledge
7) Interactive teaching style

Examples of Negative Feedback

1) Did not provide clear objectives at the start of the session and ensure these had been reached at the end. In future teaching sessions, I have implemented this and found that not only did feedback from students improve, but it gave me an objective measure of my teaching skills.

2) Slides "too wordy". I now limit myself to a maximum number of words per slide and aim that 50% of the information I present is not directly written on slides.

3) Did not involve the quieter members of the group. Although I lead very interactive teaching sessions, only certain students would actively answer questions and discuss cases. I have now changed my practice so that I ask students to discuss questions or cases in groups to ensure that they are all involved without too much pressure on individual students.

HOW DO YOU KNOW THAT YOU ARE A GOOD TEACHER?

- Positive feedback (see page 9).
- Objective measures of your teaching – students passing exams, or an objective test at the end of teaching sessions.
- Improvement in clinical practice (e.g. teaching on postpartum haemorrhage leading to an improvement in department's management of the condition).
- Students interaction with you (e.g. they appear interested).
- You are invited back to do more teaching.

TELL ME ABOUT YOUR RESEARCH EXPERIENCE

- If you have been involved in research, explain why you did it and your findings.

- If you have not been involved in research, explain any exposure you may have had to research skills and if you want to do research in the future.
    - Example 1: I have not performed any research projects, however, as a doctor I think it is extremely important to be able to critically appraise research so that an evidence-based approach can be used to provide the best care for patients. To enhance this skill, I have therefore been attending a journal club regularly.
    - Example 2: An example of where I have used evidence based medicine is...

- Be able to discuss a recent research paper (you may be asked about a research paper that has impacted your management or a recent paper that you have read).

SHOULD EVERYONE DO RESEARCH?

- It does not matter which side you favor, as long as you present well-balanced arguments for both sides and explain the pros and cons.

- NO?
  - Taking time out to do research means time out from clinical duties and if research lasts for a long time, there is a danger of losing skills.
  - Limited funding and resources for research – therefore better for more enthusiastic people to do research so as to gain maximum contribution and advancement to the field.
  - However, important to be able to understand how research is conducted and critically appraise findings.

- YES?
  - Enables doctors to better understand and appraise research papers and therefore practice evidence based medicine.
  - Contribute to medical advancement.

AUDIT VERSUS RESEARCH

- **AUDIT:** Comparing clinical practice against set standards.
- **RESEARCH:** Creating new knowledge (which may be used to develop standards).
- Therefore research establishes what the best practice should be, and audit assesses whether we are applying this best practice to our clinical activities.

Why is audit important?
- One of the seven pillars of clinical governance
- Ensures quality of care maintained at an agreed standard.
- Encourages better use of resources and improved efficiency.

Why is research important?
- Drives medical advancement by developing a pool of knowledge which can be translated into better patient care.

TELL ME ABOUT AN AUDIT THAT YOU HAVE DONE

- Explain your audit using the audit cycle:
    - Identify an issue.
    - Identify the standard.
    - Collect data on current practice.
    - Compare current practice to standards.
    - Implement change.
    - Re-audit.
    - Present the audit.

EXAMPLE:

I realised that antibiotic prescribing was not being done as well as it should be. I therefore looked up the Trust standards for antibiotic prescribing, and created a proforma with which I collected data from one hundred patients. This showed a suboptimal adherence to trust guidelines and poor documentation of the duration and reasoning for antibiotics. I presented the results at a departmental meeting and produced posters to raise awareness. A re-audit showed significant improvement, completing the audit loop.

LEADERSHIP VERSUS MANAGEMENT

- **LEADER** – sets direction/vision and directs others towards that goal.
- **MANAGER** – manages the resources to achieve it.

EXAMPLE OF LEADERSHIP AND MANAGEMENT

As a medical student, I realised how stressful final year OSCEs (Objective structured clinical examinations) can be and how important it is to identify areas of improvement early on. As a foundation year doctor, I therefore decided to organise a mock OSCE for final year medical students. This involved writing 21 scenarios and mark schemes, organising room bookings, finding patients willing to be examined and the hardest part - encouraging doctors to take an evening out of their free time to examine students. The mock-OSCE ran very well and received excellent feedback. I was awarded a leadership award for my contribution.

TELL ME ABOUT A WEAKNESS OF YOURS

- The dreaded question!!
- Use a weakness that has a positive spin and always end on a positive note.

EXAMPLE 1

I am a very enthusiastic and motivated person. This does however sometimes mean that I end up taking on too many projects at one time, which can become quite stressful and difficult to manage. E.g. Last year whilst working I was also (list other projects/activities). After reflecting on this weakness, I now make sure that I fully appreciate what other projects I have on, before undertaking new projects and if in doubt, speak to my educational supervisor.

EXAMPLE 2

I am a very caring and empathetic person. However, due to this nature, I can sometimes become too emotionally attached to patients. For example, during my last rotation, a patient who had been under our care for six weeks passed away. I found this very upsetting/distressing. When this happened, I reflected and spoke to my seniors for advice. I learnt the importance of remaining empathetic but at the same time keeping an appropriate emotional distance and I hope to develop this skill further during my training.

TELL US ABOUT A MISTAKE YOU HAVE MADE

- Ensure you discuss the following:
  - Patient safety is your priority so rectify your mistake.
  - Inform senior.
  - Be honest with patient and apologise.
  - Reflect.
  - Take steps to prevent recurrence.
    - Example 1) Discuss at teaching/departmental meetings.
    - Example 2) Make a proforma to ensure this aspect is not missed again.
  - Submit a incident report if appropriate to ensure that the hospital or department as a whole can learn from the mistake.

MBRRACE REPORT

- MBRRACE: Mothers and Babies - Reducing Risk through Audits and Confidential Enquiries across the UK

- MBRRACE is a collaboration appointed by the Healthcare Quality Improvement Partnership, which investigates maternal deaths, stillbirths, and infant deaths.

- The MBRRACE-UK Saving Lives Report is a MUST READ document for anyone applying to Obstetrics and Gynaecology Training.

- Try and bring points from the MBRRACE report into your answers.

Summary of the MBRRACE-UK Saving Lives 2015 Report:

- The MBRRACE Confidential Enquiry into Maternal Deaths report assesses maternal mortality over a three year period. The latest report was published on 8th December 2015, which looks at maternal mortality from 2011-2013.

- This report showed that maternal mortality had reduced from 11 per 100,000 to 10 per 100,000 over this time frame. Of the maternal deaths, two thirds were due to indirect causes and only one third due to direct causes.

- Indirect deaths are defined as deaths resulting from pre-existing disease, or disease that developed during pregnancy and which were not the result of direct obstetric causes, but which were aggravated by the physiological effects of pregnancy.

- Direct causes are deaths occurring from obstetric complications of pregnancy (e.g. bleeding).

- Over the last ten years, there has been a significant reduction in maternal mortality from direct causes, with a 50% decrease in deaths from direct causes over this period.

- On the contrary, there has been no significant change in the number of indirect deaths over the last ten years.

- This highlights the importance of focusing on reducing indirect deaths, by providing specialist pre-pregnancy advice, and joint specialist and maternity care.

MBRRACE-UK Saving Lives 2015 Report (Continued):

- During this triennium, causes of death in order of incidence were:
  1. Cardiac causes (indirect)
  2. Neurological causes (indirect)
  3. Thromboembolism (direct)
- Key area of improvement highlighted by the report:
  - Mental health problems
  - Drug or alcohol dependence
  - Thrombosis and thromboembolism
  - Cancer in pregnancy or postnatally
  - Domestic violence and abuse

Notes
- Nearly 1 in 5 women who died had a mental health problem.
- Women are at the higher risk of experiencing a severe (new onset) mental illness in the early days and weeks after birth than at any other time in their lives.
- Access to and uptake of antenatal care remains an issue amongst women who died. Only a third of women who died received the nationally recommended level of antenatal care.
- Although overall deaths from influenza was lower in this triennium, this is mainly due to a low level of influenza activity in 2012-2013, rather than an increase in the uptake of vaccination among pregnant women. Increasing immunisation rates in pregnancy against seasonal influenza must remain a public health priority.

MBRRACE-UK Perinatal Mortality Report

MBRRACE-UK also investigates perinatal mortality and publishes yearly reports on this subject. The last report was published on 17th May 2016, which assessed perinatal mortality from January to December 2014.

Key points:

- The extended perinatal mortality rate (from 24 weeks of pregnancy until 4 weeks after birth) in UK was 5.9 deaths per 1,000 births. This is significantly higher than rates reported in other high-income European countries.
- Therefore, there is an increasing national focus on reducing perinatal mortality with a number of national initiatives.
- These national initiatives include:
  - Each Baby Counts (The Royal College of Obstetricians and Gynaecologists - RCOG)
  - Saving Babies' Lives Care Bundle (NHS England)
  - 1000 Lives Improvement, National Stillbirth Working Group (NHS Wales)
  - Maternity and Children's Quality Improvement Collaborative (NHS Scotland)
  - The Northern Ireland Maternal and Infant Loss (NIMI) steering group
- In regards to stillbirths, 46% were due to unknown causes. This highlights an area where further assessment is required, which includes ensuring post-mortems and placental examination is offered to all bereaved mothers.

PORTFOLIO STATION MARK SCHEME

Understanding and commitment to the specialty • Why do you want to pursue a career in Obstetrics and Gynaecology? • What challenges do trainees in Obstetrics and Gynaecology face and how would you overcome these? • How have you shown commitment to the specialty? • How is Obstetrics and Gynaecology changing as a specialty? • What extra-curricular activities do you do and how will they help you in this specialty? • What is your biggest achievement and how does this apply to a career in Obstetrics and Gynaecology?	/5
Training priorities for the fist 12 months of post (and beyond) • What are your training priorities for the first 12 months and how will you achieve these?	/5
Quality improvement measures • Tell me about an audit or quality improvement project you have done? Did you close the loop/re-audit? • What is the difference between audit and research?	/5
Teaching and research experience • Have you done any research? • Do you think everyone should do research? • Tell me about you teaching experience? • How do you know that you are a good teacher?	/5
Total	/20

CLINICAL STATION

OBSTETRICS AND GYNAECOLOGY ST1
INTERVIEW BOOK

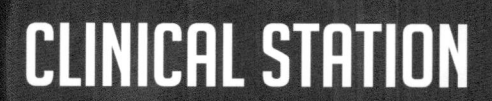

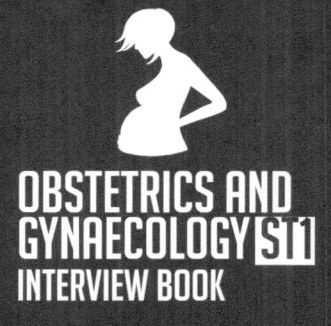

www.obsandgynae.net

CLINICAL SKILLS PRESENTATION

- In London, a prioritisation theme is followed, where you are given four to five scenarios to prioritise and manage.

- Important things to remember,
  1. Start by asking for some basic information about each patient including their observations (heart rate, respiratory rate, blood pressure, oxygen saturations, temperature) and if relevant urine dipstick and urine pregnancy test.
  2. If anyone is acutely unwell, ALWAYS seek senior help (e.g. obstetrics or gynaecology registrar/consultant, A&E consultant if in A&E, anaesthetic consultant).
  3. Think about who else can help you:
     - If a cannula is needed, do you have an FY1/nurse practitioner who you can ask to do it?
     - If a patient is pregnant but having an asthma attack in A&E, A&E or medical team can review.
     - If the patient is likely to have appendicitis, surgical team to review.

CLINICAL SKILLS SCENARIO 1

You have received the following bleeps within a 5 minute period. Please read through the scenarios below and then discuss with the examiner about how you will prioritise and manage the scenarios below.

1. 23 year old lady presenting to A&E with left iliac fossa pain.
2. 88 year old lady on the medical ward with post-menopausal bleeding.
3. 19 year old lady presenting to A&E with right iliac fossa pain and fever.
4. 48 year old lady with vaginal bleeding following a LLETZ procedure (Large Loop Excision of the Transformation Zone of the Cervix).
5. 28 year old lady who is 8 weeks pregnant with vomiting.

SCENARIO 1 – ECTOPIC PREGNANCY

1. What are her observations: "Heart rate 120, blood pressure 90/50, afebrile, respiratory rate 18, oxygen saturations 98%".

2. What are the results of her urine dipstick and urine pregnant test: "Urine dipstick negative, urine pregnancy test positive".

3. Impression: Ectopic pregnancy who is haemodynamically unstable.

4. Advise that you will come and see her as soon as possible, but in the meantime:
   - Move to A&E Resus.
   - A&E consultant/registrar to be informed.
   - Two large bore cannulae to be inserted.
   - Take bloods tests for full blood count, urea and electrolytes, clotting, group and save and a venous blood gas for an immediate haemoglobin result.
   - Cross match four units.
   - Give oxygen.
   - Initiate fluid resuscitation.

5. You will call your registrar on your way to A&E (and your consultant if you are unable to contact your registrar).

6. Whilst in A&E ensure effective fluid and blood resuscitation.

7. Recheck observations and examine (abdomen looking for signs of peritonism and speculum examination looking for bleeding).

7. Plan with registrar/consultant whether suitable for an ultrasound if stabilised or if needs to go to theatre directly.

8. If she needs to go to theatre, call porters, anaesthetist, theatre coordinator, blood bank and keep nil by mouth.

9. If very unstable may need to consider giving O negative blood whilst awaiting cross matched blood.

10. This scenario is off course your first priority.

SCENARIO 2 – POSTMENOPAUSAL BLEEDING

1. Ask why they are in hospital to start with? "Pulmonary embolism"
2. How much bleeding are they having? "Just a small amount, now resolved".
3. Observations? "Oxygen saturations 88% but otherwise normal".
4. Are they on any anticoagulation? "Yes, warfarin and low molecular weight heparin".
5. Has she had a full blood count and INR (International Normalised Ratio)? " Haemoglobin 130g/L, INR 7"
6. Impression: Stable post-menopausal bleeding, likely due to recent initiation of warfarin but need to investigate as a target patient (cancer waiting time within 2 weeks).
   - Medical team to organise a pelvic ultrasound and make a target referral to the gynaecology rapid access clinic.
   - Unlikely to appear in interviews but if post-menopausal bleeding is very heavy and unstable, will need urgent review, speculum +/- tranexamic acid.

SCENARIO 3 – APPENDICITIS

1. What are her observations?: "Heart rate 120, blood pressure 100/50, temperature 39, respiratory rate 18, oxygen saturations 98%".
2. What are the results of her urine dipstick and urine pregnant test?: "Urine dipstick negative, urinary pregnancy test negative"
3. Any previous operations? "No"
4. Impression: Most likely appendicitis and she is septic.
5. Management: Ask A&E team to move to A&E Resus, perform the Sepsis Six care bundle and to refer urgently to surgeons.

SCENARIO 4 – BLEEDING POST-OPERATIVE FROM A LLETZ PROCEDURE

1. Check observations and amount of bleeding : "Obs stable and minimal bleeding".
2. You can ask if the doctor who performed the procedure is available to review. If not, when you review you will examine and cauterise any bleeding points with silver nitrate. Ask the nurse to inform you in the interim if there is any increase in bleeding or if her observations become unstable.

SCENARIO 5 – HYPEREMESIS GRAVIDUM

1. What are her observations?: "Obs all stable".

2. Has she had a urine dipstick and pregnancy test?: "Urine dipstick shows 3+ ketones. Urinary pregnancy test positive".

3. Management:

• Admit (Generally we admit patients with more than 2+ ketones in their urine or patients who are unable to keep down any oral intake or with significant weight loss).

• Perform blood tests for full blood count, renal function and electrolytes, liver function tests (and thyroid function tests if recurrent hyperemesis).

• Ensure intravenous access, intravenous fluids (including treatment of any electrolyte imbalance).

• Prescribe antiemetics, ranitidine, vitamin replacement (thiamine, folic acid).

• Remember thromboprophylaxis.

• Arrange an ultrasound to look for multiple/molar pregnancy.

4. Note: Vomiting in pregnancy is common. However, not all vomiting in pregnancy is hyperemesis gravidum.

OTHER COMMON SCENARIOS

SCENARIO 6 - POST-OPERATIVE SEPSIS
- "A 32 year old lady attends A&E five days after having had a Caesarean section feeling generally unwell. How would you manage her?"

- Observations? "Temperature 38.5, blood pressure 110/86, heart rate 110, respiratory rate 16, oxygen saturations 100% on air."
- Observations suggest she is SEPTIC therefore inform A&E consultant/anaesthetist and move her into Resus.
- Carry out the sepsis six care bundle (blood cultures, full blood count and lactate, oxygen, intravenous fluids, catheterise and measure urine output).
- Take bloods for renal function, electrolytes and C-reactive protein.
- Take a full set of cultures including mid stream urine, vaginal swab, throat swab, MRSA (methicillin resistant staphylococcus aureus) swabs and swabs from all surgical site.
- Organise a chest x-ray.
- Inform registrar/consultant.
- Full assessment: Look at throat, listen to chest, examine breasts, palpate abdomen (examine wound site, is uterus well contracted)?, speculum examination and swabs, evaluate lochia and examine legs (pulmonary embolism can cause raised temperature).
- Empirical antibiotics depending on allergies: cefuroxime and metronidazole are broad spectrum and safe in breastfeeding but check hospital protocol or can ask senior/microbiologist for advice.
- Consider further imaging (ultrasound or CT scan).
- Potential sources of infection: Endometritis, retained products of pregnancy, urinary tract infection, chest sepsis, mastitis.

SCENARIO 7 - POST-OPERATIVE BLEED
- "You are called to the ward to see a lady who is bleeding heavily six hours post-operatively from an abdominal myomectomy. How would you manage her?"

- What are her observations? "Heart rate 110, blood pressure 100/65, afebrile, 100% on air, respiratory rate 18".
- What is her urine output? "20ml in the last hour"
- Pre-op haemoglobin and estimated blood loss? "120g/L, estimated blood loss 1L"
- Was it a complicated surgery? "Dense adhesions"
- Drain output? "200ml in the last 2 hours"
- Tell the nurse you will come immediately, but in the meantime would she be able to ensure that the patient has two large bore cannulae and take bloods for full blood count, group and save and a venous blood gas for an immediate haemoglobin. Instruct the nurse to initiate a 1L bag of Hartmann's STAT.
- "On your arrival, repeat observations are blood pressure 90/60, heart rate 130 . Venous blood gas shows haemoglobin 65g/L. She now has 600ml in the drain."
- Urgently call registrar/consultant and anaesthetist as the patient likely needs to go to theatre. Ask the nurse to call theatre, porters, blood bank and cross match four units. If there is a delay in receiving blood (e.g. not already group and saved, ask for O negative blood).
- Whilst awaiting senior support, quickly assess the abdomen for signs of peritonism as well as the drain and wound sites for bleeding.

SCENARIO 8 - POST-OPERATIVE PAIN

— "You are called to see a 52 year old lady day zero post abdominal hysterectomy complaining of abdominal pain."

- What are her observations? "All stable"
- Any bleeding? "No"
- Drain output? "15ml in 4 hours"
- Urine output? "200ml in 4 hours"
- What analgesia is she on? "Paracetamol only"
- As she is clinically stable, you can ask your FY1 to assess and prescribe analgesia (and to inform you if further concerns).

SCENARIO 9 - OVARIAN CYST ACCIDENT

-"28 year old female attends A&E with right iliac fossa pain and vomiting. How would you manage?"

- Observations: "Heart rate 110, blood pressure 120/80, afebrile".
- Urine dipstick and urinary pregnancy test?: "Negative"
- Any operations in the past? "Appendicectomy"
- Any diarrhoea? "No"
- Impression? Ovarian cyst accident
- Ask A&E team to ensure she has intravenous access, send bloods including full blood count, renal function and electrolytes, C-reaction protein, group and save and venous blood gas for lactate. Ask A&E team to give analgesia, intravenous fluids and antiemetics.
- Full assessment on your arrival including abdominal examination, vaginal examination and speculum including swabs. Inform your senior urgently as may be ovarian cyst torsion.
- If clinically there are signs of peritonism or severe pain and vomiting – may need to take woman to theatre prior to ultrasound due to concern about torsion. Otherwise offer urgent ultrasound. But this needs discussion with a senior!
- If for theatre,
    - Inform anaesthetist, theatre co-ordinator and porters.
    - Ensure full blood count, group and save and intravenous access.
    - Complete consent form and keep nil by mouth.

SCENARIO 10 - PELVIC INFLAMMATORY DISEASE

- "23 year old lady attends A&E with left iliac fossa pain"
  - Observations: "Heart rate 120, blood pressure 110/81, temperature 39, oxygen saturations 100 percent, respiratory rate 16".
  - Urine dipstick and urine pregnancy test: "Negative"
  - Impression: ? Pelvic inflammatory disease or pyelonephritis (less likely with negative urine dipstick). However, she is septic and needs urgent attention.
  - Plan:
    - Move to A&E Resus.
    - Inform anaesthetist/A&E consultant.
    - She is septic so needs resuscitation including sepsis six care bundle (blood cultures, full blood count and lactate, catheterise and monitor urine output, oxygen, intravenous fluids and intravenous antibiotics).
    - In addition, take bloods for urea and electrolytes and C-reactive protein.
    - Take a full set of cultures including mid stream urine, high vaginal and endocervical swab and consider a chest x-ray.
    - Inform senior.
  - History:
    - Urinary/bowel symptoms
    - Gynaecological history
    - Risk factors for pelvic inflammatory disease (sexual history, use of intrauterine coil, previous pelvic surgery).
  - Examine: chest, abdomen, speculum (including triple swabs) and vaginal examination (may elicit cervical excitation and adnexal tenderness).
  - Arrange ultrasound scan to look for free fluid/tuboovarian abscess.

CLINICAL SCENARIOS (OUTSIDE OF LONDON)

Outside of London, you are only dealing with one scenario, so you have to approach it in a more detailed manner.

EXAMPLE 1:
The Brief

A 21-year-old college student presents with 2 days of vaginal spotting and lower abdominal discomfort. Her last menstrual period was approximately 5 weeks ago, and her only past medical history is of pelvic inflammatory disease. She is not on any medications and has no known drug allergies. She is a smoker. Her vital signs are heart rate 110, blood pressure 90/50, temperature 37 degrees celcius, oxygen saturations 97%, respiratory rate 12. On examination she is tender in the right iliac fossa with guarding and has brown vaginal discharge.

How would you manage this case?

- Don't just say ABC! Explain yourself.

- "I will introduce myself to the patient and confirm her details. This will allow me to know she is alert and her airway is patent. If she is stable enough I will take a quick history."

- "I will then do a complete physical examination including abdominal and speculum with a chaparone. I will send endocervical and high vaginal swabs." The examiner informs you that she is tender in the right iliac fossa with guarding. She also has some brown vaginal discharge.

- "I will ask for a urine dipstick and urine pregnancy test."

- "As she is tachycardic and hypotensive, I will insert two large bore cannulae (grey) and take bloods for full blood count, renal function, group and save, and cross match 4-6 units. I will prescribe and give 1 litre intravenous fluid STAT."

- "I would do urine dipstick to look for signs of a urinary tract infection and a urinary pregnancy test. I would like to know if there has been any drop in her haemoglobin which would be suggestive of an internal bleed (e.g. ruptured ectopic pregnancy). I would like to know her white cell count to see if there is evidence of infection. I would order group and save in case she needs a blood transfusion or surgical management."

- "I would admit the patient and inform my seniors. I would also organise an ultrasound of the pelvis if she is stable."
- Examiner: "The patient has deteriorated now and become more tachycardic with a pulse of 125 and hypotensive with a blood pressure of 80/50. The urine pregnancy test is positive, urine dipstick is negative. Haemoglobin on a venous blood gas is 75g/L but the other blood tests are awaited. How would you proceed?"
- "My differential diagnosis is an ectopic pregnancy. She is already being resuscitated, so I would like to inform my registrar immediately as they can do a bedside scan and look for free fluid in the pelvis."
- Examiner: "Your registrar is in a room doing an instrumental delivery."
- "Then I would like to talk to my consultant, because this patient will likely need to go to theatre as I suspect she may have a ruptured ectopic."
- Examiner: "The consultant will be here in 20 minutes. What would you like to do now?"
- " I will prepare the patient for theatre. I will give her another litre of fluid and call the blood bank to ensure she has been cross matched 4-6 units. If there is a delay in receiving blood and the patient is unstable, I will consider giving O negative blood. I will inform the anaesthetist and theatre staff. I will find and fill out a consent form, ready for the consultant's arrival."
- Examiner: "The consultant is here, what do you say?"
- Give a comprehensive handover...
- To impress them even more and if you have time left, tell them:
- I will consent her for laparoscopy+/-laparotomy +/- salpingectomy/ salpingotomy.
- Complications: bleeding, infection, injury to surrounding structures, (bowel, bladder, ureters, large blood vessels), thromboembolic disease.
- Other procedures: Repair of any damage, blood transfusion.

EXAMPLE 2:
The Brief
As an ST1, you are called to see a patient one day following laparoscopic assisted vaginal hysterectomy. She is hypotensive and tachycardic. On examination you find her abdomen rigid with guarding and rebound tenderness. Your registrar is "scrubbed up" in theatre and cannot respond.

What do you do next?
- State that you will attend to the patient straight away.
- Perform ABCDE.
- Ask for vital signs: "blood pressure 100/50, heart rate 120, respiratory rate 14, oxygen saturations 97%, temperature 36.6 degrees celsius")
- Ask about urine output ("15ml/hour").
- Ask about drain output (100ml in drain over 2 hours)
- Ask about vaginal pack (soaked)
- Examine (rigid abdomen with guarding and rebound tenderness)
- Resuscitate - intravenous access (x2 grey cannulae), URGENT bloods for full blood count, renal function and electrolytes, C-reactive protein, group and save and cross match 4-6 units.
- Do a venous blood gas and find out the pre-operative haemoglobin.
- Give intravenous fluids and oxygen.
- Check the drug chart: Has she been prescribed adequate analgesia?
- Read the operation notes: From the operation notes you will find that the operation was challenging due to adhesions and haemostasis was difficult to achieve.
- Examiner: "The venous blood gas shows her haemoglobin is 74g/L. It was 125g/L pre-operatively".
- Tell them that you suspect a post operative internal bleed, and therefore the patient will likely need to go back to theatre.
- Inform the gynaecology registrar if available or the on call consultant. If both are busy, you can speak to the obstetric consultant/registrar or the consultant who performed the surgery.
- Prepare the patient for theatre: Call blood bank, theatre team, anaesthetist, porters and consent the patient if you are able to.

CLINICAL MOCK INTERVIEW STATION 1

You have received the following bleeps within a 5 minute period. Please read through the scenarios below and then discuss with the examiner about how you will prioritise the scenarios below.

A. 21 year old lady presenting to A&E with right iliac fossa pain.

B. 23 year old lady presenting to A&E with left iliac fossa pain and a known left sided ovarian cyst.

C. 92 year old lady on the acute medical unit with a single episode of vaginal bleeding.

D. 48 year old lady who is day 0 post abdominal myomectomy feeling generally unwell.

E. An episiotomy requiring repair on labour ward.

CLINICAL MOCK INTERVIEW STATION 1 - ANSWERS

Rapid assessment and prioritisation	/3
Appropriate management of Ms A: • Observations: Heart rate 110, temperature 38, respiratory rate 18, oxygen saturations 98%, blood pressure 128/72. • Investigations: urine dip and pregnancy test negative. • Impression: Likely appendicitis but septic. • Management: Ask A&E to refer to surgeons but whilst awaiting surgical review for A&E team to perform septic screen (full blood count and lactate, intravenous fluids and antibiotics, blood cultures, measure urine output).	/3
Appropriate management of Ms B: • Observations: Heart rate 120, blood pressure 90/60, respiratory rate 22, afebrile. • Investigations: Urine dip 2+ blood, urinary pregnancy test positive. • Impression: Most urgent, likely ectopic pregnancy. • Management: Inform seniors (registrar/consultant) and involve anaesthetist/A&E consultant as unstable. Move to A&E resus, and resuscitate (provide oxygen, ensure two large bore cannulae from which take blood for full blood count, group and save (and cross match four units) and a venous blood gas for immediate haemoglobin. Give intravenous fluids/blood transfusion. Catheterise and monitor urine output). • If stabilises, consider ultrasound scan. If unstable, will likely need to go to theatre. In that case, liase with theatre co-ordinator, porters, blood bank and anaesthetist and consent patient if you are able to. • Consider O negative blood if unstable.	/5
Appropriate management of Ms C: • Observations: Stable, minimal bleeding. • Investigations: Full blood count done – haemoglobin 12g/L, International Normalised Ratio (INR) 8 on warfarin. • Impression: Post-menopausal bleeding, not acute but needs referral as target (cancer pathway). • Management: Ask medical team to arrange ultrasound and gynaecology outpatient follow up as target.	/3
Appropriate management of Ms D: • Observations: Stable, good urine output, 20ml in drain, minimal blood loss in theatre, not on any pain killers. • Management: Ask FY1/anaesthetist to assess and prescribe analgesia.	/3
Appropriate management of Ms E: • Observations: Pulse 88, blood pressure 130/80, minimal active bleeding. • Impression: Stable. • Management: Ask if midwife can suture.	/3
Total	/20

CLINICAL MOCK INTERVIEW STATION 2

You have received the following bleeps within a 5 minute period. Please read through the scenarios below and then discuss with the examiner about how you will prioritise the scenarios below.

A. 19 year old lady presenting to A&E with right iliac fossa pain and fever.

B. 33 year old lady with prolonged menstrual bleed.

C. 48 year old lady with vaginal bleeding following a LLETZ procedure (Large Loop Excision of the Transformation Zone of the Cervix).

D. A cannula required on the gynaecology ward for a patient with hyperemesis.

E. 23 year old lady presenting to A&E with left iliac fossa pain.

CLINICAL MOCK INTERVIEW STATION 2 - ANSWERS

Rapid assessment and prioritisation	/3
Appropriate management of Ms A: • Observations: Heart rate 110, temperature 38, respiratory rate 18, blood pressure 115/67. • Investigations: Urine dipstick and pregnancy test negative. • Impression: Likely appendicitis but septic. • Management: Ask to refer to surgeons but whilst awaiting surgeons for A&E team to do septic screen (lactate, bloods, blood cultures, mid stream urine, intravenous access, antibiotics, intravenous fluids).	/3
Appropriate management of Ms B: • Observations: Heart rate 80, blood pressure 130/62, temperature 37, respiratory rate 16, oxygen saturations 100 percent. • Investigations: Urine dip 3+ blood, urinary pregnancy test negative, haemoglobin on venous blood gas 128g/L. • Management: Check smear status, examine (abdomen, speculum and swabs), send full blood count, could consider a course of norethisterone and ask GP to refer to gynaecology outpatients.	/3
Appropriate management of Ms C: • Observations: Blood pressure 120/60, heart rate 70, afebrile, minimal bleeding. • Management: Ask nurse to see if doctor who performed procedure is available. When you review, examine and cauterise any bleeding lesions with silver nitrate.	/3
Appropriate management of Ms D: • Observations stable. • Management: Ask FY1/site nurse manager to cannulate.	/3
Appropriate management of Ms E: • Observations: Temperature 38, heart rate 110, respiratory rate 22, blood pressure 95/62, oxygen saturations 100 percent. • Investigations: urinary pregnancy test negative, urine dipstick negative. Haemoglobin 120g/L, white cell count 28, C-reactive protein 320. • Impression: Pelvic Inflammatory disease. Unlikely pyelonephritis in view of negative urine dipstick. • Management: Septic – therefore resuscitate and perform sepsis six (full blood count and lactate, blood cultures, intravenous access, fluids and antibiotics, oxygen, catheterise and monitor urine output). Inform senior and inform anaesthetist as acutely unwell. Transfer to A&E resus. Examine including vaginal examination, speculum and triple swabs (cervical excitation on examination, and left adnexal tenderness).	/5
Total	/20

CLINICAL MOCK INTERVIEW STATION 3

You have received the following bleeps within a 5 minute period. Please read through the scenarios below and then discuss with the examiner about how you will prioritise the scenarios below.

- A. 27 year old lady with heavy bleeding two weeks after a Caesarean section.
- B. 30 year old female who is 24 weeks pregnant with back pain and rigors.
- C. 32 year old lady in A&E who is 14 weeks pregnant with a history of asthma and is complaining of severe shortness of breath.
- D. 18 year old lady in A&E with right iliac fossa pain.
- E. 65 year old in the acute assessment unit with an abdominal mass.

CLINICAL MOCK INTERVIEW STATION 3 - ANSWERS

Rapid assessment and prioritisation	/3
Appropriate management of Ms A: • Observations: Heart rate 130, blood pressure 72/48, temperature 36, respiratory rate 22, oxygen saturations 100 percent on air. • Investigations: Urine dipstick: blood +++ • Impression: UNSTABLE. Haemorrhagic shock secondary to ? retained products of conception/chorioamnionitis. • Management – Inform seniors and anaesthetist/A&E consultant. Move to A&E resus. Ensure two large bore cannulae, intravenous fluids, oxygen, bloods including full blood count, group and save and venous blood gas for immediate haemoglobin. Cross match four units. • Present venous blood gas to examinee and ask them to interpret - pH 7.28, Pco2 7, Hco3- 18, base excess -4 lactate 3, haemoglobin 90 • Explain that the venous blood gas shows a) signs of anaemia secondary to haemorrhage and b) metabolic acidosis and raised lactate likely secondary to haemorrhagic shock/sepsis. • The patient's temperature spikes to 39 degrees – How would you manage now? • Perform sepsis 6 including intravenous antibiotics, intravenous fluids, blood cultures, mid-stream urine, swabs, urinary catheter and monitor urine output. Ensure senior aware. Consider ultrasound to look for retained products of conception +/- evacuation of retained products of conception (ERPC) to remove source of infection and haemorrhage.	/5
Appropriate management of Ms B: • Observations: Temperature 38, blood pressure 130/84, heart rate 88. • Investigations: Urine dipstick: leucocytes 3+ nitrites + protein +. • Impression: Likely pyelonephritis. • Management: If FY1 is available, can ask them to see – prescribe intravenous fluids, intravenous antibiotics, analgesia, send of bloods and septic screen and inform obstetric registrar.	/3
Appropriate management of Ms C: • Observations: Respiratory rate 32, oxygen saturations 88%, heart rate 110, blood pressure 130/88. • Impression: ? flare of asthma/PE/other cause – acutely unwell. • Management: Needs to be seen urgently but ask A&E consultant to manage and move to resus! Explain acute management of asthma safe in pregnancy.	/3

CLINICAL MOCK INTERVIEW STATION 3 - ANSWERS

Appropriate management of Ms D: • Observations: Heart rate 88, blood pressure 120/80, temperature 37.8. • Investigations: Urine dipstick negative. Urine pregnancy test negative. Blood tests pending. • Impression: Most likely appendicitis. • Management: Ask surgical team to review and to discuss with you if gynaecological review is required.	/3
Appropriate management of Ms E: • Observations stable, afebrile • Management: Ask medical team to arrange target (two week wait) ultrasound and gynaecology outpatient follow up. You will ask your day team to review in the morning.	/3
Total	/20

CLINICAL MOCK INTERVIEW STATION 4

You have received the following bleeps within a 5 minute period. Please read through the scenarios below and then discuss with the examiner about how you will prioritise the scenarios below.

- A. 77 year old lady on the medical ward with post-menopausal bleeding.
- B. 27 year old lady who is feeling unwell 2 days after a Caesarean section.
- C. Missing drug chart on a ward for a patient who is due to have their antiepileptic medications.
- D. 16 year old lady with right iliac fossa pain.
- E. 22 year old lady in A&E with a vulval haematoma following a tight rope accident.

CLINICAL MOCK INTERVIEW STATION 4 - ANSWERS

Rapid assessment and prioritisation	/3
Appropriate management of Ms A: • Observations: Heart rate 80, blood pressure 142/88, afebrile. • Investigations: Haemoglobin 110g/L, not on warfarin. • Impression: Post-menopausal bleeding but stable. • Management: Ask medical team to arrange ultrasound and gynaecology follow up as target (cancer pathway). Will review when free/ask day team to review.	/3

Appropriate management of Ms B:
• Observations: Blood pressure 130/80, heart rate 120, oxygen saturations 88% on air, respiratory rate 22, afebrile.
• Other bedside information: Good urine output, minimal blood in drain.
• Investigations: Not had any yet.
• Impression: Pulmonary embolism
• Management:
  • Needs urgent assessment.
  • Investigations: Electrocardiogram (sinus tachycardia), arterial blood gas (p02 8, pCO2 4, pH 7.25, HCO3- 25, lactate 3), bloods (haemoglobin 110g/L, white cell count 8, C-reactive protein 20, D-dimers raised, normal renal profile), chest x-ray (normal), ventilation perfusion scan (V/Q) /CT pulmonary angiogram (CTPA) - results pending.
  • Treatment: Oxygen, intravenous access, inform senior and anaesthetist/medical team. Consider starting treatment dose low molecular weight heparin pending results of scan.
	/5

Appropriate management of Ms C: • Management: Ask FY1 to prescribe anti-epileptics as does need to be given on time.	/3
Appropriate management of Ms D: • Observations: Temperature 39, blood pressure 120/80, heart rate 120. • Investigations: Urine dipstick and pregnancy test negative. • Impression: Likely appendicitis but septic. • Management: Ask to refer to surgeons but whilst awaiting surgeons for A&E team to do septic screen (lactate, bloods, blood cultures, mid stream urine, antibiotics, intravenous access and fluids, catheterise and monitor urine output).	/3
Appropriate management of Ms E: • Observations: Heart rate 88, blood pressure 120/80, afebrile. • Other information: Not actively bleeding. • Investigations: Urine dipstick and urinary pregnancy test negative • Management: Ask nurse to take bloods for full blood count and give analgesia and icepack whilst awaiting review).	/2
Total	/20

CLINICAL MOCK INTERVIEW STATION 5 (WITH ANSWERS)

Part 1: You have been called to see Mrs Smith, a 28 year old female who has attended A&E with left iliac fossa pain.

Talk me through your assessment, differentials, investigations and management.

Assessment and Investigations: • Observations (stable) • Introduction • History (including SOCRATES, history of bleeding/shoulder tip pain/ syncope, risk factors for ectopic pregnancy, sexual history, urinary/ bowel symptoms). • Physical examination (abdominal, vaginal examination, speculum) • Blood test (full blood count, renal function and electrolytes, C-reaction protein, group and save). • Urine dipstick (negative) and urine pregnancy test (positive). • Inform senior. • Organise an urgent ultrasound scan.	/7
Differentials • Ectopic pregnancy (until proven otherwise) • Urinary tract infection/pyelonephritis • Diverticulitis • Renal colic	/3

Part 2: Whilst you are organising an ultrasound scan, the nurse calls you to say her blood pressure has dropped and is now 93/56. Her heart rate is now 120. What are your revised differentials?

Differentials • Likely ruptured ectopic.	/3

What would you do next?

Management	/7
<ul><li>Use ABCDE approach.</li><li>Obtain intravenous access and fluid resuscitate.</li><li>Send off full blood count, venous blood gas (haemoglobin 6g/L) and cross match four units. Consider O negative blood.</li><li>Insert catheter to monitor urine output.</li><li>Move to Resus.</li><li>Inform A&E consultant and gynaecology registrar/consultant.</li><li>Will likely need to go to theatre for ruptured ectopic pregnancy (inform anaesthetist, porters, theatre co-ordinator).</li></ul>	

How would you consent this patient for surgery?

<ul><li>Laparoscopy +- salpingostomy +- salpingectomy</li><li>Bleeding</li><li>Infection</li><li>Damage to nearby structures (bladder, bowel, ureters, blood vessels)</li><li>Thromboembolic disease</li><li>Anaesthetic risks</li><li>If salpingostomy, will need further monitoring and rarely further procedure.</li><li>Other procedures: blood transfusion, laparotomy, repair of any damage, oophrectomy</li></ul>	/5
Overall clinical aptitude	/5
Total	/30

CLINICAL MOCK INTERVIEW STATION 6 (WITH ANSWERS)

Part 1: You are an FY2 and called by a nurse on the gynaecology ward. There is a 49 year old lady who is day 2 post abdominal hysterectomy. She has started complaining of pain in her abdomen. Her observations are blood pressure 90/50, heart rate 120, temperature 38.5 degrees celcius.

Assessment and Investigations: • ABCDE approach • Resuscitate (2 large bore cannulae, arterial blood gas for lactate, full blood count, urea and electrolytes, C-reactive protein, coagulation screen, group and save, oxygen, catheter to monitor urine output and intravenous fluids). • Blood cultures and intravenous antibiotics. • Wound swabs, mid stream urine, high vaginal swab. • Full examination (chest, abdomen, speculum and swabs). • Inform seniors including anaesthetist.	/6
Differentials • Sepsis secondary to wound infection or intra-abdominal infection/collection.	/3
What is sepsis? • Systemic Inflammatory Response Syndrome (SIRS): • Temperature >38 or <36 • Heart rate >90 • Respiratory rate >20 or an arterial partial pressure of carbon dioxide less than 4.3 • White cell count >12 or <4 • Sepsis is SIRS due to an infective cause.	/5

Her arterial blood gas shows:

pH 7.22, pCO2 2.2, pO2 12, HCO3 18, Lactate 5, Base Excess -8

Explain the findings and suggest an initial management plan:

<ul><li>Metabolic acidosis with partial respiratory compensation.</li><li>Lactate >4 is a sign of severe sepsis.</li><li>Patient needs fluid resuscitation.</li><li>Monitor response to fluids by monitoring urine output, blood pressure and repeat venous blood gases.</li><li>If not already informed, seniors should be called.</li><li>If does not respond to fluid challenge, this is septic shock and she needs Intensive Therapy Unit (ITU) for inotropes.</li></ul>	/5

What is the definition of severe sepsis and what features may be associated with it?

• Severe sepsis refers to sepsis-induced tissue hypoperfusion or organ dysfunction.	/2
• Clinical features include reduced Glasgow Coma Scale (GCS), hypotension, oliguria, mental status changes, prolonged capillary refill time and cool, clammy skin.	/2
• Investigation findings include raised creatinine suggesting acute renal injury, raised lactate, deranged clotting, deranged liver function tests, raised haematocrit, evidence of disseminated intravascular coagulation (prolonged prothrombin time and activated partial thromboplastin time, raised D-dimer, low fibrinogen), and metabolic acidosis.	/2
Overall clinical aptitude	/5
Total	/20

COMMUNICATION STATION

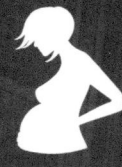

OBSTETRICS AND GYNAECOLOGY ST1
INTERVIEW BOOK

www.obsandgynae.net

COMMUNICATION STATION

- Although this is named the "communication station", do not be fooled. It tests a combination of clinical and communication skills.

- General advice:
  - Scenarios are designed to be realistic, therefore remain calm and act as you would in reality – If you were called to see this patient, what would you do?
  - Would you want to know their observations? If the answer is yes, then ask for them.

    e.g. "We are just going to put a small monitor on your finger and a blood pressure cuff on your arm just to check a few of your measurements."
  - Would you want an electrocardiogram (ECG)?

    e.g. "We are going to put some leads on your chest to measure the activity of your heart."
  - Scenarios are very repetitive – practice previous scenarios!
  - Use non-medical terminology.
  - Introduce yourself and your role at the start of the consultation and offer follow-up at the end.
  - Give information in bite-sized pieces and check for understanding.

PULMONARY EMBOLISM

- **HISTORY** – Ensure you take a full history of the pain (use SOCRATES mnemonic). Ask about associated symptoms (including cough, fever, calf pain, shortness of breath, palpitations, dizziness), risk factors for pulmonary embolism (recent travel/surgery, immobilisation, fractured bones, use of combined oral contraceptive pill, personal or family history, smoker).

- **EXAMINATION** – Ask for observations, perform a cardiac/respiratory exam and examine calves.

- **INVESTIGATIONS** – Bloods (full blood count, C-reactive protein, D-dimer), arterial blood gas, electrocardiogram (ECG), chest-Xray, ventilation perfusion scan (V/Q scan)/CT pulmonary angiogram (CTPA).

- **OXYGEN** – In the history, if the patient states that they are short of breath, say "I am just going to put an oxygen mask on you to help you breathe."

- **MANAGEMENT** – Ask if they want anyone in the room when you explain the diagnosis and further management. Explain that the shortness of breath may be due to a clot in the lungs. You will start them on a blood thinning injection to prevent spread of any clot until further imaging.
- Patient may ask, "Will I be okay Doctor?"
  - Example answer: It's a good thing you came into hospital and we have picked this up early. If picked up early like in your case, and treated properly, it is unlikely to cause any significant long term problems. However, we do need to keep you in hospital and keep a close eye on you at the moment.

PULMONARY EMBOLISM STATION (2) - ANGRY PATIENT

"You are a different doctor. The patient comes to see you as they are upset about being sent home without advice regarding INR monitoring on warfarin. This led to them having a significant nose bleed."

APOLOGISE
- Listen. Allow the patient time to express their concerns.
- Apologise for the distress caused.

INVESTIGATE
- Plan to obtain notes and review these with a senior to assess how care could have been improved.
- Put in an incident report, which goes to the management team who will investigate the case.
- Consider organising teaching or bringing up the issue at the next departmental meeting to bring about awareness and prevent recurrence.
- Offer the patient details of Patient Advice and Liason Service (PALS) if they want to put it an official complaint.

FOLLOW UP
- Offer the patient a follow up meeting to discuss the outcome of any investigation.
- Is there anything else we can do to help you?

GENERAL MEDICAL CARE
- How is the patient otherwise? How is their recovery and how are their symptoms?
- If complaint is about lack of explanation regarding condition and management, explain this to them and provide a leaflet.

ANGRY PATIENT

USEFUL PHRASES

- "I apologise for the distress this has caused you. It is important that we investigate it thoroughly so that we can take steps to prevent it happening in the future."
- "Doctors and nurses would never intentionally give suboptimal care. I'm sure my colleague would appreciate this feedback and I will definitely pass it along to him/her."
- "I'm sorry you feel like you have not been given the information you need."

ANAEMIA DUE TO MENORRHAGIA

- **HISTORY**
  - History of menorrhagia (need for double protection, any clots, flooding).
  - Symptoms of anaemia (shortness of breath, dizziness, fatigue).
  - Effect on quality of life.
  - Menstrual cycle (age at menarche, regularity of cycles, how long bleeds are, intermenstrual/postcoital bleeding, dysmenorrhoea, dyspareunia).
  - Gynaecological history (smear results, contraception, any previous sexually transmitted infections).
  - Obstetric history (parity and outcome of any pregnancies).
  - Exclude other potential sources of bleeding.
    a) History of presenting complaint (any rectal bleeding, malaena, weight loss, night sweats or haemoptysis which could suggest gastrointestinal, respiratory or malignant cause).
    b) Medication history (use of steroids/non-steroidal anti inflammatory drug could predispose to peptic ulcer).
    c) Recent surgery (post-operative bleed).
    d) Social history (alcohol and cirrhosis suggestive of variceal bleed).

- **EXAMINATION**
  - Ask for observations and perform a full examination. You may then be told that relevant findings include a heart rate of 120 and a palpable fibroid uterus.

- **COUNSELING FOR BLOOD TRANSFUSION**
  - Counsel regarding
    - Type of blood products
    - Indication for transfusion
    - Benefits and risks
    - Possible alternatives (e.g. iron infusion)
    - How transfusion is administered
  - Inform patient that following a blood transfusion they can no longer be a donor.
  - Give written information.
  - Check if patient needs time to consider/any further information.

ANAEMIA DUE TO MENORRHAGIA

- **RISKS OF BLOOD TRANSFUSION**
  - Viral Infections
    - HIV: 1 in 6 million
    - Hepatitis: 1 in 1 million
    - Hep C: 1 in 72 million
  - Allergic or immune reaction: common
  - Anaphylaxis/immune reaction: serious but rare
  - Development of antibodies

EXAMPLE ANSWER

- The reason you are feeling tired and short of breath is because you have a low red blood count. We suspect this is because of the heavy bleeding you have been having.
- We would recommend a blood transfusion, where we put a drip into your arm and replace those blood cells, which will make you feel better.
- Blood transfusions are fairly common. The risk of serious side effects is low. There is a small risk of infection, but all blood donors are carefully selected and tested for infections to ensure blood donated is as safe as possible. The risk of hepatitis or HIV is less than 1 in a million.
- Some people who have a blood transfusion can have an allergic reaction. This is usually just a little bit of itching and we can give you tablets to help with that. Rarely, you could have a severe allergic reaction.
- There is a risk of your body reacting to the blood products by producing antibodies. Antibodies are small protein molecules that circulate in the blood and recognise certain molecules as foreign. This may make it more difficult to obtain compatible blood if you require transfusion in the future.

ANAEMIA DUE TO MENORRHAGIA

- You will be regularly monitored whilst having the blood transfusion and immediately after it. This includes checking your blood pressure, heart rate and pulse. If you develop any signs of having a reaction, we would stop the transfusion straight away and start any necessary treatment.

- **ALTERNATIVES**
    - Iron tablets – Iron is a component of red blood cells. Iron tablets slowly increase blood levels over the next six to eight weeks. Side effects include constipation and vomiting.
    - Iron infusion – Increases iron levels over 2-3 weeks. Small risk of allergic reaction.
- Ask if they have any questions and if there is anything else you can advise them about to help make their decision.
- Give a leaflet.

PELVIC INFLAMMATORY DISEASE

- **HISTORY**
  - "I will need to ask you some personal questions. Everything you say is confidential and any information you provide will help to work out what is causing your pain so we can treat you effectively."
  - If any discharge, ask about colour, itchiness, odour.
  - Any pain or irregular bleeding?
  - When was her last sexual intercourse? Regular or casual partner? Male or female? Type of sex?
  - Any history of sexually transmitted infections?
  - Contraception use?
  - Previous pregnancies?

- **EXAMINATION**
  - "I am going to put a probe on your finger and a cuff around your arm to get some basic measurements. We will also measure your temperature. I am then going to feel your tummy and do an internal examination and take some infection swabs. Would this be okay? Nurse Emma will be here as a chaperone and we will lock the door to ensure your privacy."

- **INVESTIGATIONS**
  - "We need to do some blood tests to look at your infection markers. Would that be okay? We also need to test your urine for infection and to test for a pregnancy. We will also organise a ultrasound scan of the tummy."

- **DIAGNOSIS AND MANAGEMENT**
  - Say that you are going to explain the diagnosis and management. Does she want anyone in the room with them whilst you go through it?
  - "The pain you are having is most likely due to an infection in the womb and tubes. We call this pelvic inflammatory disease."
  - "The infection is treated by giving you a course of antibiotics for 14 days. It is very important that you complete the course even if you are feeling better as if you stop part way through the course, the infection can recur, resulting in complications."

PELVIC INFLAMMATORY DISEASE

- "As this may be due to a sexually transmitted infection, it is important that you refrain from sexual intercourse or use barrier contraception such as condoms whilst you are on treatment. You should attend a sexual health clinic and have a sexual health screen after the treatment is complete, to ensure that the infection has cleared."
- "It is also important that your partner is treated regardless of what screening shows. Most males are asymptomatic and screening only picks up about half of cases. If any partners have the infection and it is not treated, the infection will pass back and forth."
- "We advise that you inform any partners that you have had in the last six months, so that they can receive the appropriate treatment and prevent long-term complications. The sexual health clinic can do this for you if you prefer."

- **LONG TERM COUNSELING**
  - "There are some potential long term consequences of this condition. These risks increase with recurrent episodes of this condition, therefore, it is important you take steps from preventing a recurrence."
  - "These complications include long term pain, difficulty getting pregnant and pregnancies occurring outside the womb and in one of the tubes known as ectopic pregnancies."
  - "To prevent this happening again, it is important to use condoms. It is important to know that whilst other forms of contraception prevent pregnancies, they do not prevent sexually transmitted infections. It is also important to have regular sexual health checks if you have a new partner or symptoms such as abnormal vaginal discharge or pain in your tummy."

BREAKING BAD NEWS: MISCARRIAGE

The Brief
- A 32 year old lady has been having vaginal bleeding and abdominal cramping for the last few days.
- She has just had a pelvis ultrasound scan which shows a missed miscarriage at 6 weeks.
- Please see the patient and explain the ultrasound results.

HOW TO MANAGE

Introduction and history
- Introduce yourself & your role
- Make sure she is stable enough for a discussion (i.e. observation stable).
- Set the scene (go to a quiet room, switch off your bleep).
- Ask the patient if there is anyone she would like to call.
- Take a quick history (SOCRATES for pain, volume of bleeding, dizziness, shoulder tip pain, obstetric and gynaecological history including last menstrual period and outcome of any previous pregnancies, last smear test, history of sexually transmitted infections, any other medical/surgical/drug history or allergies.

Breaking Bad News
- Ascertain prior knowledge (what does she already know?)
- Give warning shots ("I am afraid it is not good news")
- Explain the ultrasound report:
  - Be clear ("You have had a miscarriage")
  - Don't waffle
  - No jargon
  - Don't give false hope
- Pause! Allow her the opportunity to cry and provide her tissues if she does.
- Be sympathetic but professional.

Further Information
- Once she has calmed down, give her some statistics:
  - It is NOT HER FAULT!
  - Miscarriages are very common (1 in 4).
  - Most miscarriages are one off (sporadic).
  - Chances of a future healthy pregnancy is the same as someone who has not had a miscarriage.
  - Most common cause is chromosomal abnormality in the fetus. No investigation unless three consecutive miscarriages.
  - No treatment to prevent miscarriage.
- Further management:
  - If the miscarriage is complete- no further treatment.
  - If the miscarriage is incomplete- give her further management options.

HOW TO MANAGE

Further management options

1) Letting nature take its course (expectant management)
   - Successful in 50% of women.
   - Bleeding and cramping can last up to 3 weeks.
   - If severe bleeding and pain, may need emergency admission.
2) Taking tablets (medical management)
   - Successful in 85% of women.
   - Medication allows neck of the womb to open and pregnancy tissue to pass.
   - Usually takes hours to days to work during which she can experience pain and heavy bleeding. Pain relief and anti-sickness tablets will be provided.
   - Can go home after tablet administered. However, if heavy bleeding may need admission.
3) Having an operation (surgical management)
   - Successful in 95% of women.
   - Done under general anaesthesia.
   - The neck of the womb is gently opened and pregnancy tissue is removed using a suction device. The procedure is called Surgical Management of Miscarriage (SMM).
   - It is a commonly performed operation and generally safe. However there is a small risk of complications (bleeding, infection, incomplete procedure and need for further intervention, uterine perforation). The risk of uterine perforation (making a hole in the uterus) is 5 in a 1000 but if this occurs, there is a risk of damage to structures in the tummy including bowel, bladder, tubes that go to the bladder (ureters) and blood vessels. In the event that the uterus is perforated, laparoscopy (keyhole surgery) or laparotomy (cut in the tummy) may be needed to check for/repair any damage.
   - The risk of infection is the same for surgical and medical management.

Ending the consultation

- Check her understanding.
- Ask if she has any questions.
- Acknowledge that you have given her a lot of information.
- Ask if she wants to go and think about the options.
- Offer her a second appointment once she has made a decision.
- Offer leaflet.
- Seek medical advice urgently if heavy bleeding, pain not relieved with analgesia, offensive smelling vaginal discharge or flu-like symptoms such as shivers or raised temperature.

CHLAMYDIA IN AN ANGRY PATIENT

The Brief

- A 30 year old patient with a one week history of abnormal vaginal discharge was seen last week in clinic and has come back to find out the results of her triple swabs and ultrasound.
- The ultrasound is normal, however, the swabs show that the patient has chlamydia.
- The patient has being waiting for 30 minutes.
- Please see the patient and inform her of the results.

HOW TO ANSWER

Introduction and dealing with an angry patient
- Read the brief carefully (you are 30 minutes late!)
- Don't be fooled - this scenario is also a breaking bad news station.
- Introduce yourself and your role.
- Be prepared, the patient will be ANGRY!
- Listen to her and don't interrupt!
- APOLOGISE PROFUSELY!
- Explain to her that you were late because you were attending to another emergency.
- Offer her discussion with a more senior doctor.
- Offer her the contact details for Patient Advice and Liason Service (PALS) if she remains angry.
- Never raise your voice.
- Remain calm, apologetic and sympathetic.

Breaking Bad News
- Recap, "I understand you've being having some discharge and had an ultrasound and some swabs taken. How are you feeling now?"
- Give the good news first, the ultrasound is NORMAL.
- "But I am afraid the swab results show you have chlamydia."
- Pause!
- "However, it is easily treated with antibiotics."

Further Information
- Give her some information, SLOWLY, don't regurgitate everything you know. Avoid jargon.
  - Chlamydia is a sexually transmitted infection.
  - It is common amongst young people.
  - It is easily treated with oral antibiotics.
  - You can catch chlamydia when you have unprotected sex with someone who already has the infection. This can be by vaginal sex, oral sex or anal sex.

HOW TO ANSWER

Long term complications and further management
- Tell her about future complications
  - Chlamydia is unlikely to lead to any long-term problems if it is treated quickly. However, without treatment chlamydia can cause serious problems.
  - Women can develop pelvic inflammatory disease (PID). This can cause abdominal and pelvic pain. It can also lead to sub-fertility (difficulty getting pregnant) and ectopic pregnancy (a pregnancy that occurs outside the womb).
  - In rare cases, chlamydia may cause other symptoms such as arthritis (swollen joints) and inflammation of the eyes. (This is known as Reiter's syndrome and is more common in men).
- Further advice
  - "You should avoid any sex, even with a condom, until after both you and your partner have finished your treatment."
  - "You need to ensure you are tested to ensure the infection has gone after you complete treatment. You can do this at any sexual health clinic, and I can provide you with details of these."
  - "If you have chlamydia, you should also be tested for other sexually transmitted infections such as HIV, syphilis, hepatitis B and gonorrhoea, as you can have more than one infection at the same time."
- Know the importance of **contact tracing**! "It is essential that your current sexual partner, and any other sexual partner you have had over the last six months, are tested and treated. This is to stop you getting the infection again, and also to prevent your partners developing any complications."

Ending the consultation
- Offer to answer any question she may have.
- Give an imaginary leaflet!
- Apologise again for being late!

DEEP VEIN THROMBOSIS IN A 15 YEAR OLD

The Brief

You have admitted a 15 year old girl to the hospital with a diagnosis of deep vein thrombosis. She started taking the oral contraceptive pill 6 months ago, which was prescribed by the GP.

She is an occasional smoker. She has no past medical history. She currently had a boyfriend with whom she is sexually active. <u>She has given you permission to discuss any details of her condition with her parents,</u> but warns you that her father is "very old fashioned" and is not aware that she is on the pill or that she is sexually active.

Please speak to her parents.

HOW TO ANSWER

Introduction
- Introduce yourself and your role
- Check understanding (how much does the father know?)
- Reassure the father that his daughter is clinically stable.
- Give warning shots! "There are a few different issues that I need to discuss with you, some of which might come as a surprise to you."

Clinical Explanation
- Explain DVT in simple terminology
  - "Blood clot in the leg, restricting blood flow."
- Explain immediate treatment
  - "We have started your daughter on an injection that thins the blood. This will prevent more blood clots from forming."
- Explain long term management
  - "We will also need to start your daughter on another type of medication called warfarin. This will also work by thinning the blood and she will need to remain on it for at least 3 months. She will need regular monitoring of her blood clotting ability during this period."
- Explain any complications
  - "At the moment, things are under control, but if the blood clot dislodges it can travel to her lungs and cause problems with her breathing which can be serious."
- Do not overstate danger!
- "Long term problems are unlikely. However your daughter will be considered high risk for blood clots and hence in the future she may need to take precautions when taking long haul flights or deciding to get pregnant."

HOW TO ANSWER

Reasoning for PE

- "Why did this happen?"
  - Explain the risk factors for deep vein thrombosis.
  - "The majority of blood clots happen for no reason, but there are few things that make it more likely for someone to develop blood clots, for example taking the oral contraceptive pill or smoking."
  - If asked, state that the patient had two risk factors, oral contraceptive pill and smoking.
- Patient's father may become angry, in which case:
  - Apologise and acknowledge.
  - " I understand that some of this information may come as a surprise to you, I am sorry if that makes you feel upset."
- He may ask who started the contraceptive pill and how it was possible to without his consent:
  - Inform him that it was started by the GP.
  - Explain about Gillick competence.
  - "It is legal for doctors to prescribe medication for underage patients if they are able to understand the implications and effects of the medications."
  - "This is also done because it is preferable for teenagers to be using birth control and protection than having unprotected sexual intercourse because of fear that the information will be revealed to their parents."

Angry patient and completing the consultation

- The patient's father remains angry and wants to complain:
  - Apologise and remain calm.
  - Acknowledge it is a lot of information to take in.
  - Give him the opportunity to speak to a senior member of staff.
  - Give information about PALS (Patient Advice and Liason Service).
  - Give him a leaflet on deep vein thrombosis.

COMMUNICATION MOCK INTERVIEW STATION 1

INSTRUCTIONS BEFORE ENTERING
You are the Senior House Officer in Accident and Emergency. Your next patient has been waiting a long time to see you. She has presented with chest pain. Please take a history, ask for relevant examination and investigation findings, and explain the diagnosis and treatment to the patient. You will be stopped at half time.

HISTORY
You are a 23 year old female who has had sharp pain under her left breast since yesterday evening. Paracetamol does not relieve the pain. The pain is worse on taking a deep breath in. You have coughed up some fresh blood this morning. You are a smoker and are on the oral contraceptive pill (do not state unless specifically asked). You have never had a pulmonary embolism or deep vein thrombosis before. Your mum had a 'blood clot in her lungs'. You are not pregnant. No recent travel/surgery/fracture.

EXAMINATION
- Chest – clear
- Heart sounds – normal
- Respiratory rate – 32
- Heart rate – 120
- Oxygen saturations – 96% on air
- Temperature – 37.0
- Left calf – red and painful

INVESTIGATIONS
- Chest x-ray – normal
- Electrocardiogram – sinus tachycardia
- Troponin – negative
- D-dimer – positive
- Arterial blood gas – signs of respiratory alkalosis with mild hypoxia
- CT pulmonary angiogram – shows pulmonary embolism

SECOND HALF OF SCENARIO
Stop candidate. Scenario moves forward 3 days. Patient has been admitted to hospital for treatment of her pulmonary embolism. She has now written a formal letter of complaint as she feels that there has been poor communication with her.

MARK SCHEME FOR COMMUNICATION MOCK INTERVIEW STATION 1

Introduces self, grade	/2
Listens to patient ideas, concerns and expectations	/2
History taking • History of presenting complaint including assessment of pain and associated symptoms (shortness of breath, cough, calf pain) • Risk factors for thromboembolic disease	/4
Examination • Observations • Chest exam • Leg exam	/3
Investigations • Chest X-ray • Bloods including D-dimer • Electrocardiogram (ECG) • CT Pulmonary Angiogram (CTPA)/Ventilation Perfusion Scan (V/Q)	/3
Management • Offers analgesia and oxygen • Treatment dose low molecular weight heparin pending investigations • Need for warfarin for at least 3 months	/3
Breaking bad news • Asks patient what she knows • Breaks news gently • Explains diagnosis in simple terms	/2
Managing an angry patient and complaint • Listens to and empathises with patient's concerns • Apologises to patient • Explores events with patient • Offers patient opportunity to talk to a senior • Offers patient contact details of PALS if she wishes to take this further	/4
Patient score	/3
Examiner score	/4
Overall score	**/30**

COMMUNICATION MOCK INTERVIEW STATION 2

INSTRUCTIONS BEFORE ENTERING
You are the Senior House Officer in Accident and Emergency. Your next patient has presented with lower abdominal pain. Please take a brief history, ask for relevant examination and investigation findings, and explain the diagnosis to the patient. You will be stopped at half time.

HISTORY
You are a 19 year old female who has a history of lower abdominal pain and deep dyspareunia. This has been ongoing for two months, but has become unbearable over the past 24 hours. You have purulent vaginal discharge but no nausea or vomiting. You have no urinary or bowel symptoms. You broke up with your long term partner three months ago, and have had unprotected sexual intercourse with a new partner since then. Your periods are irregular and your last period was 3 weeks ago. You have never been pregnant.

EXAMINATION
- Chest – clear
- Heart sounds – normal
- Abdomen – diffuse lower abdominal tenderness
- Respiratory rate – 16
- Heart rate – 76
- Oxygen saturations – 100% on air
- Temperature – 38.5
- Pelvis – cervical excitation and bilateral adnexal tenderness

INVESTIGATIONS
- Urinary pregnancy test - negative
- Bloods – raised white cell count and C-reactive protein, otherwise normal
- Endocervical swab – chlamydia

SECOND HALF OF SCENARIO
Stop candidate. Scenario moves forward 4 weeks. The patient has returned to hospital. You are a different doctor. She is concerned that she believes the doctor she saw previously was rude, and led her to believe she will be infertile.

MARK SCHEME FOR COMMUNICATION MOCK INTERVIEW STATION 2

Introduces self, grade	/2
Listens to patient ideas, concerns and expectations	/2
History taking • History of presenting complaint - including assessment of pain, discharge and deep dyspareunia • Sexual history	/4
Examination • Observations • Abdominal examination • Pelvic examination	/3
Investigations • Urinary pregnancy test • Full blood count, C-reactive protein • Triple swabs	/3
Management • Assesses patient's current understanding • Breaks news gently • Explains diagnosis in simple terms • Explains importance of contact tracing • Explains importance of barrier contraception to reduce further risk • Explain possible long term effects (subfertillty, ectopic pregnancy, chronic pain)	/3
Managing an angry patient • Listens to and empathises with patient's concerns • Apologises to patient • Explores events with patient • Offers patient opportunity to talk to a senior • Offers patient contact details of PALS if she wishes to take this further	/6
Patient score	/3
Examiner score	/4
Overall score	**/30**

COMMUNICATION MOCK INTERVIEW STATION 3

INSTRUCTIONS BEFORE ENTERING:
You are the Senior House Officer in A&E. Your next patient has presented with severe fatigue with a full blood count showing a haemoglobin of 62g/L. Please take a history, ask for relevant examination findings, and explain the diagnosis and treatment to the patient.

HISTORY
You are a 35 year old female who has been feeling tired all the time for the past few months. You have also been feeling short of breath on exertion. You have heavy periods, changing your pad up to every hour during the first few days, with clots and flooding. You have a thirty day regular cycle with seven days of bleeding. You use condoms for contraception, and do not think you could be pregnant. You have no other past medical history. Your smear tests are up to date and normal.

EXAMINATION
- Respiratory rate – 16
- Heart rate – 104
- Oxygen saturations – 99% on air
- Temperature – 37.2
- Chest – clear
- Heart sounds – normal
- Abdomen – soft but with a palpable fibroid uterus

MARK SCHEME FOR COMMUNICATION MOCK INTERVIEW STATION 3

Introduces self, grade	/2
Listens to patient ideas, concerns and expectations	/2
History taking • Symptoms of anaemia • History of menorrhagia (how heavy is the bleeding, need for double barrier protection, presence of clots, flooding) • Menstrual history (regularity of cycle, how long bleeds last for, presence of inter-menstrual or post-coital bleeding) • Gynaecological history (smear history, sexual history, contraception) • Obstetric history (outcome of any pregnancies) • Other potential causes of bleeding (haematemesis, malaena, night sweats, weight loss, swollen glands, recent surgery)	/4
Examination • Observations • Abdominal examination	/3
Management • Discusses need for investigation of heavy menstrual bleeding with an ultrasound scan • Discusses need for management of anaemia in the acute situation (see below)	/3
Consent for a blood transfusion • Explains reason for transfusion • Explains benefits of a blood transfusion • Explains risks of a blood transfusion (infection, allergic reaction, anaphylaxis, development of antibodies) • Explains alternatives to blood transfusion (iron tablets and infusion) • Explains what blood transfusion will involve (staying in hospital, cannula, close observation) • Asks if patient has any questions • Offers written information and time to make a decision	/6
Patient score	/3
Examiner score	/4
Overall score	**/30**

COMMUNICATION MOCK INTERVIEW STATION 4

INSTRUCTIONS BEFORE ENTERING:
You are the Senior House Officer in Gynaecology. Your next patient has presented with heavy vaginal bleeding. Please take a history, ask for relevant examination and investigation findings, and explain the diagnosis and treatment to the patient.

HISTORY
You are a 28 year old female with a 4 hour history of heavy vaginal bleeding and associated mild lower abdominal crampy pain. You are 10 weeks pregnant. You have been changing pads every 15-30 minutes and the bleeding is getting heavier. You are feeling very weak. You have had 1 previous termination of pregnancy and no previous sexually transmitted infections. You have not had an ultrasound in this pregnancy. You have no other past medical or surgical history.

EXAMINATION
- Respiratory rate – 20
- Heart rate – 120
- Blood Pressure – 90/60
- Oxygen saturations – 99% on air
- Temperature – 37.0
- Chest – clear
- Heart sounds – normal
- Abdominal exam – soft, non-tender
- Speculum – cervical os open with heavy vaginal bleeding

INVESTIGATIONS
- Urinary pregnancy test – positive
- Haemoglobin – 80g/L (previously 120g/L)

MARK SCHEME FOR COMMUNICATION MOCK INTERVIEW STATION 4

Introduces self, grade and role	/2
Listens to patient ideas, concerns and expectations	/2
History taking • History of presenting complaint including assessment of severity of bleeding • Symptoms of anaemia: dizziness/shortness of breath • Risk factors for ectopic pregnancy (previous abdominal operations/ sexually transmitted infections, smoking, intrauterine coil devices)	/4
Examination • Observations • Abdominal examination • Pelvic examination	/2
Investigations • Haemoglobin • Group and save/cross match • Urinary pregnancy test	/2
Management • Resuscitate (cannula, intravenous fluids) • Consider blood • Senior support	/2
Breaking bad news • Explain to patient that she is miscarrying • Breaks news gently • Explains in simple terms	/3

Consent for "Surgical Management of Miscarriage (SMM)"
• Explains what procedure is
• Explains reason for procedure
• Explains how the procedure is performed
• Explains risks of procedure
  • General (bleeding and need for blood transfusion, infection, pain, thromboembolic disease)
  • Specific (uterine perforation and damage to nearby structures which could require laparoscopy/laparotomy and repair of damage, incomplete procedure and need for repeat procedure)
• Asks if patient has any questions
	/6

Patient score	/3
Examiner score	/4
Overall score	**/30**

Printed in Great Britain
by Amazon